Living
Beyond
Grief

Dr. Roy W. Harris

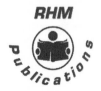

Recommended by Others

Living Beyond Grief by Dr. Roy Harris offers practical steps of application for those experiencing the devastation of losing a loved one. I read several books after losing my parents, but this book has given me new insights in helping me as I journey through the grieving process. I highly recommend this book to those on this same path of grief.

PAMELA S. HACKETT

Pam is a pastor's wife to her husband Tim, a mother and grandmother. She experienced first hand the loss of both of her parents and the grief that comes with such a great loss. She's also been front and center for countless others as they've navigated the difficult journey of grieving.

Living Beyond Grief is very readable, practical, and helpful, whatever your situation. Roy takes us through his deepest journey as though we were passengers strapped in for the ride, and from scene to scene we gain new insights. Who knew a book about caregiving, grief, and recovery could be so enriching and — should I say it? — Entertaining.

Dr. ROBERT J. MORGAN

Rob has served as pastor of The Donelson Fellowship for over 30 years. He is a best selling and Gold-Medallion winning writer of over 40 books with over 3.5 million books in print circulation.

Can anyone fully understand the many emotions a caregiver goes through in the loss of a loved one? From his experience, Roy Harris poignantly shares practical insights on grieving and healing in his book *Living Beyond Grief.* There's nothing quite like hearing from someone who's been there and is thriving. Share this book with someone who is working through his or her own grief! **SANDY ATWOOD**

Sandy is a wife, mother and grandmother. She has faithfully stood by her pastor husband Richard as they've both experienced great personal loss of family members. She is also a writer and editor for Randall House Publications.

About the Author

Roy Harris is a husband, father, grandfather, pastor, an educator and published author. He faithfully stood by his wife of 33 years Diana through their three-year battle with breast cancer that eventually took her life.

His book *Caring for the Caregiver* has been used mightily by God across America and the world helping and encouraging caregivers. It also provides insight to family members, pastors and friends into what caregivers experience. The book is now available in 24 countries around the globe.

His latest book *Living Beyond Grief* is a sequel written to help those who've lost loved ones navigate the difficult waters of grief.

Roy has successfully with God's help, moved through those difficult days and not only survived but is doing well.

God had a plan for Roy's life that

included *living beyond his grief*. God brought a wonderful rainbow named Amy into his life that became his best friend, partner in ministry and helpmate.

Roy couldn't have imagined the great things God had in store for him in his future *after grief*.

He came to understand that nothing takes God by surprise. That everything that happens to God's children is always for their good and His glory.

Roy holds Bachelor of Arts and Master of Ministry degrees from Welch College and a Doctor of Philosophy degree from Trinity Theological Seminary. He's spoken in over 400 churches, civic organizations, educational institutions, and other venues.

He's a minister, conference, seminar and retreat speaker having spoken in 38 US states, Kenya, Tanzania, Uganda, Rwanda, Europe and Israel.

Roy is and published author with 14 books in print including four in Swahili.

Contents

Introduction

I slowly walked from the graveside to my car numb from all that had taken place over the past three days.

I left Harris Chapel Cemetery with the emptiest feeling deep down inside that I'd ever experienced in my life.

My thoughts went to my children Missy and Aaron and the fact they had just lost their mother much earlier in life than normally happens. To Glenn and Kathleen Thomas who lost a daughter and Diana's siblings who lost a sister.

We gathered at the Cookeville Free Will Baptist Church for a delicious meal. The children made the 50-mile trip back to the Nashville, TN area and I spent the night with my parents in Cookeville.

I was glad not to be alone. Exhausted, I

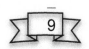

was surprised how soon the sun came up and another day had dawned. What would this day be like?

Merriam Webster's Dictionary defines grief as *deep and poignant distress caused by bereavement.* The Cambridge Dictionary describes it as *very great sadness* and the English Oxford Dictionary defines it as *intense sorrow, especially caused by someone's death.*

Grief brings deep sorrow and mental distress caused by loss, remorse or affliction. Grief is an emotion that is a normal part of life.

The word grief means pain or sorrow over a loss that hurts deeply. It is a life changing emotion and it can be a life shattering emotion.

Grief may generate other emotions like fear, anger, resentment, worry and guilt.

Grief may manifest itself in a variety of ways such as loss of sleep, loss of appetite and loss of self-control.

However one might define it, grief is

one of the most painful emotions and periods of grief are some of the most difficult times we face in life. How we handle grief will impact our immediate and long term happiness.

Decisions made during periods of grief can unknowingly create barriers to future hope and happiness.

It is possible to not only survive grief but also to thrive on the other side of grief.

The following pages record one man's journey through the grieving process and also encouragement and advice for others who may be traveling down a similar road.

Dr. Roy W. Harris

Death is Approaching

Almost three years had passed since we first began the difficult journey. It had been obvious that Diana's future did not look good. The fluid build up around her lungs had subsided and doctors determined that the tube implanted months before was no longer necessary. They felt it should be removed and the opening closed to lesson the possibility of infection. This would not be a difficult procedure but a little risky because of her weakened physical condition.

The operation was scheduled a few days later at Baptist Hospital. The surgery was performed and pronounced successful by the same surgeon who implanted the tube earlier.

This was becoming almost a routine. So many procedures, so many hours in waiting rooms before, during and after surgeries – but this time would be drastically different. I was not ready for what I was about to hear.

The surgeon entered the waiting room and I asked him how Diana was doing, meaning did she come through the surgery okay. His response caught me completely by surprise. He said, "She is dying. She is not the same lady I saw a few months back when we implanted the drainage tube. She has declined drastically."

I was completely numb. I am not completely sure of the exact wording of the entire conversation. I mumbled asking, "How long does she have to live?"

He responded: "maybe two months at the most."

Deep down I knew this day might come but I was not ready for it. I do not remember much after that. My mind was running in so many directions. How would I tell Diana? The kids would need to be told. Diana's parents would need to know.

The things that lay ahead seemed too hard to contemplate. But I had no choice. The family looked to me for strength and leadership. I knew I must somehow determine who should know, what order and when. I'd promised Diana that I wouldn't keep bad news from her. How and when should I tell her? Diana's sister, Dorene, was with us and heard my conversation with the doctor.

Diana's parents had already planned to spend a few days with us and would arrive the next day. I thought it over and decided Saturday evening would be the best time to inform the family. Diana was sleeping much of the day now. I would wait until she went to bed and then deliver the difficult news to the family.

The next couple of days seemed so long. I rehearsed how I would tell the family and changed the wording over and over in my mind. Saturday evening finally arrived. I prayed and asked God to guide my thoughts and give me words that would convey the necessary bad news, and still have an underlying strength that would give a sense of God's peace and presence.

Diana retired early. The men were upstairs and the ladies downstairs. We could not all congregate upstairs and leave Diana alone downstairs, and we could not all gather downstairs fearing that Diana might be awakened and overhear the conversation.

Dorene told the ladies as I was telling the men. There were looks of shock and tears of sadness. We consoled each other as best we could. Dorene agreed to tell the rest of Diana's side of the family and I would tell my side.

It was done... With one huge hurdle crossed, my thoughts began to drift again toward the week to come. How would I tell Diana? She'd asked me only a few weeks before if I thought she was going to "make it." How could I find the words? How could I keep my composure? How would she take it? How and when would be the best time?

Hearing the news that your loved one is going die is devastating. Many people only think of grief occurring after loved ones have passed on.

There is much more to it. Grieving actually begins when caregivers, family members and friends realize that things are never going to be the same again. They also realize that the person they care for is going to die. The grieving process begins with the anticipation of what is soon to occur. This initial part of grief is called *anticipatory grief*.

Grief generates a number of stages through which caregivers must pass. Grieving may begin long before the actual death of the loved one. If the illness is long term with gradually declining heath, anticipating the approaching loss of a loved one can begin long before they actually pass away.

Anticipatory grief, as it sometimes referred to, is the grief caregivers experience when they recognize that the loss of a loved

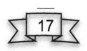

one or friend will happen in the future but it has not actually yet happened (Erickson, 2012)

Anticipatory grief is absent from many grief models. However it is an important part of the grieving process. Anticipatory grief provides an opportunity for loved ones and caregivers to prepare for the end they know is coming.

This preparation could include seeking forgiveness, finalizing family affairs and making plans with loved ones about their impending exit from this life (Ibid).

Anticipatory grief normally creates emotional highs and lows bringing up and down periods on the emotional roller coaster for caregivers.

Dr. Elisabeth Kubler-Ross created the Grief Cycle Model first published in *On Death & Dying* in 1969, which has commonly been used to describe feelings of both unpaid family care providers and those receiving care.

Although every situation is different, most caregivers will pass through at least one or more of the stages of Kubler-Ross's grief model. They will experience many of the feelings mentioned in her model (Kubler-Ross, 1969).

Dr. Elisabeth Kubler-Ross' Grief Cycle model includes these five stages:

1. Stage I: *Denial*. A good definition by Kubler-Ross of denial is a conscious or unconscious refusal to accept facts, information, reality, etc., relating to the situation concerned. She suggests that denial is a defense mechanism and perfectly natural.

There is real danger here. Some people can become locked into this stage when dealing with a traumatic change, which they choose to ignore. We know that death is not easy to avoid or hide from indefinitely.

2. Stage II: ***Anger***. Kubler-Ross suggests that anger can be manifested in different ways. People who are dealing with emotionally upsetting events can become angry with themselves and/or with others but especially those close to them.

This is important to remember for friends and families of caregivers. This will help them better understand what is happening and keep a detached and non-judgmental attitude when experiencing the anger of caregivers who have entered the grieving process.

3. Stage III: ***Bargaining***. Traditionally, people facing death or realizations that the death of a loved one will probably occur do the bargaining stage of grief.

An attempt is made to make a deal with God in exchange for one's own life or the life of a loved one. People facing less serious trauma than death often bargain or seek to negotiate a compromise with God. Bargaining rarely provides a sustainable solution, especially if it's a matter of life or death.

People make promises to God to begin some things or cease from doing others if God will heal the loved one or friend.

4. Stage IV: **Depression**. Kubler suggests that depression is often referred to as *preparatory grieving*. She describes it as the dress rehearsal or the practice run for the things that are coming.

This stage means different things depending on whom it involves. It begins with the acceptance of what may be coming without the full emotional attachment that it will require.

It is natural to experience the emotions of sadness, regret, fear, uncertainty and many others. When caregivers reach this stage, they have begun to accept the reality of the loss that is about to happen or already has happened.

5. Stage V: **Acceptance**. This stage definitely varies according to the caregiver's situation. Kubler-Ross suggests that in a broad way, this stage is an indication that there is

some emotional detachment and objectivity on the part of the caregiver.

People dying can enter this stage long before the caregivers they leave behind, but caregivers must also pass through their own individual stages of dealing with their grief.

Anticipatory grief can impact the family caregiver in a number of ways but the three most common ways are physically, emotionally and spiritually.

According to Kubler-Ross, the caregiver may experience a number of grief symptoms during anticipatory grief (Kubler-Ross, 1969). These include but are not limited to:

1. Physical symptoms of anticipatory grief may include the following:
   a. Low energy
   b. Exhaustion
   c. Headaches
   d. Upset stomach
   e. Sleeping more than usual
   f. Pushing themselves to extremes

at work

2. Emotional symptoms of anticipatory grief may include:

    a. Memory gaps

    b. Preoccupation

    c. Irritability

    d. Depression

    e. Euphoria

    f. Rage

    g. Passive resignation

    h. Imitate loved ones feelings

3. Spiritual symptoms of anticipatory grief may include:

    a. Feel closer to God than the past

    b. Outrage towards God

    c. Feel cut off from God and wondering where He is

    d. Temporary paralysis of one's spirit

Remember, there is hope for the believer, even during this difficult period of anticipating what may be coming.

The term *hope* is not mentioned by Dr. Kubler-Ross but is important especially for a person with faith in God. HOPE moves the caregiver through each stage to the *ultimate hope*, which is *eternal life*.

David Cowles suggests the value of hope and how it may be reflected in the five stages of Kubler-Ross' grief model (Cowles, 2003).

Hope found by Cowles in the Kubler-Ross model is reflected below:

1. Stage I: **Denial**. The *HOPE* is to find a second opinion or to have further tests to verify an accurate diagnosis and prognosis.
2. Stage II: **Anger**. The *HOPE* is to find a cure, seeking other treatment options, healing and remission of the disease process.
3. Stage III: **Bargaining**. The *HOPE* is for more time to complete personal goals in

the immediate future.

4. Stage IV: **Depression**. The *HOPE* is for less discomfort and maximum pain relief for the loved one.

5. Stage V: **Acceptance**. The *HOPE* is for family support and preparation for the end of this life and transition to eternal life.

Georgia Shaffer reflected on her grief journey. "Looking back it was my relationship with God, my friends, and the psychologist that gave me hope to continue; God took all that was lost and used it to transform my life." (Shaffer, 200, p. 27)

Psalm 3:2-6 says, *Many are saying of me, God will not deliver him. But you, LORD, are a shield around me, my glory, the One who lifts my head high. I call out to the LORD, and he answers me from his holy mountain. I lie down and sleep; I wake again, because the LORD sustains me. I will not fear though tens of thousands assail me on every side.*

GRIEVING PRINCIPLE: Do not lose hope! Hope in the Lord will sustain and deliver you during this difficult time. Hold on to it.

When The Death Angel Comes

I dreaded the ride home. What could I say? How could I encourage her? She had just heard that she would die soon. I was truly amazed with what took place.

Diana was more upbeat than she had been in a year. She knew the kids were coming over and she was excited about seeing them and the grandchildren. Her appetite had waned but now she had a craving for pizza from Pizza Hut.

I had arranged for the entire family to eat supper together that evening. The kids knew their mom would find out about her impending death by the oncology doctor that day and we all wanted to be together to comfort her and support each other.

Diana laughed and played with the grandchildren. It was one of the most enjoyable evenings we'd had in a long time. She stayed up later than normal and seemed to have a burst of energy not present for months.

Shortly after midnight I was awakened by Diana's need to be helped to the restroom. I lifted her from bed and placed her in the wheelchair, taking care to position the oxygen line so we could make it easily to the restroom.

I helped her get situated and left the room with the door cracked to give her some privacy. She cried out and I quickly ran and opened the door. *I cannot feel my legs*, she said.

I was not overly alarmed because of previous times when her leg or arm would go to sleep. I helped her back into the wheel chair and back to the bed. I began to rub one leg and then the other to get circulation moving again.

Dorene was sleeping lightly and awoke to something happening downstairs. She came into the room and I told of the numbness. She began to help me rub Diana's legs. In a few moments Diana's parents heard the moans of pain and the frantic efforts to bring some relief to her aching legs. They joined us and it became obvious that the situation was not improving.

I called 911 and requested an ambulance. The paramedics arrived within minutes and determined she needed to be transported to the hospital. Dorene agreed to ride with Diana in the ambulance and I would drive Diana's parents and myself.

We arrived a few minutes before the ambulance and waited at the door of the ER as Diana arrived. Diana's parents remained in the waiting area, and Dorene and I stayed with Diana.

After the examination, the doctor wanted to talk with me outside the room. I will always remember the conversation that followed.

The doctor began his diagnosis. Diana had developed a blood clot in the main artery that delivered blood flow to her lower extremities.

There was no blood flowing to her legs. I stood there stunned. I couldn't think. I remember asking him what it meant and what could we do?

He replied, *"She is going to die. We could do surgery, but she is in such bad shape that she will not survive open-heart surgery."*

I asked him if there was anything we could do? He said they would make her as comfortable as possible and that nothing else could be done. He said she would probably not live through the night.

What should I do now? Diana's parents were in the waiting area. They needed to know.

The children needed to know so they could spend those last few hours with their mother.

Her siblings should know.

My parents, my brother and his family and my church family needed to know. My head was spinning. I knew deep down this day might come. I never dreamed it would arrive so quickly.

Dorene and I walked to the waiting area and sat down with Diana's parents. I tried to speak as tenderly and compassionately as I could.

I repeated the diagnosis and told them the doctor said Diana was not going to make it.

The sadness in their eyes was beyond description. Dorene sat with her parents and tried to give them comfort.

I could not sit long. The children needed to know. I did not want to give them such sad news on the phone. I stepped outside the ER into the night air and called both children. I told them to come to Baptist Hospital as soon as they could, that things did not look good for their mother.

Diana had not been told how serious things were. I felt as if the weight of the whole world was on my shoulders.

How could I tell her she was about to die? I was about to lose the person who had been the love of my life for the past thirty-three years. I just could not be the one to do it.

I asked the doctor to wait until the children arrived to tell Diana. We gathered beside her bed as the doctor walked in.

He got Diana's attention and began to tell her of the blood clot and what was happening to her body. He told her nothing could be done and that she would not make it.

My son broke down in the room. There were tears all around and a feeling of helplessness. We could do nothing but yet we had to do something.

Eventually it was determined that it would be better to move Diana from the ER to a private room and make her as comfortable as possible.

A male nurse accompanied us as we made our way to the elevator, down a long hallway to the assigned room.

We almost lost Diana in the hallway but the nurse was able to revive her. We eventually made it to a room around daybreak.

Diana took a turn for the better that would last most of the day. It didn't take long for word of her impending death to run the circuit throughout the city.

All who knew her loved her, and there was a continual flow of friends through Baptist hospital.

The day became more difficult as the minutes passed. It would be twenty-two hours from the first alarm until the final goodbye.

It's hard to describe what was going through my mind. Physically I was so tired. It had been over a year since I'd slept an entire night.

I could sense the end was near for a

relationship that had begun over thirty-four years ago.

My thoughts were not of the past or the future but making sure she did not suffer. Her death would come softly and peacefully.

The technicians placed a hand held *pain relief pump* at Diana's side. Pain relief medicine could be injected directly via I.V. into her bloodstream every fifteen minutes.

The doctors were amazed at how she was able to survive and remain conscious when her lower extremities were dying.

I sat by her bedside, across the room, on the windowsill, leaving the room only briefly a few times. I had such mixed feelings. She had suffered so much with this terrible disease.

Death was near. Selfishly, I could not imagine life without her but I did not want her suffering to continue.

My emotions moved into a feeling of numbness. I was involved with something I had absolutely no control over.

God creates life and all life belongs to Him. The circle of life ends where it begins, in the hands of God. The circle of Diana's life on this earth was about to be completed.

The day continued to move forward, mid-morning, noon, 3:00 p.m. About 6 p.m. Diana slowly drifted into unconsciousness. She lay there for three to four more hours.

The room, hallway, and waiting area were filled with family, friends, co-workers and church members. Many had been with us for several hours.

I'm not sure of the exact time, but around 9:30 p.m. one of the most unusual things happened that I have ever witnessed.

Diana awoke. She was completely awake. She sat up quickly in the bed gazing toward the ceiling.

She had a glow about her that is impossible to adequately describe. She reached her arms toward Heaven as if reaching to embrace someone.

It was as if no one else was in the

room. It was obvious she saw a heavenly being who was about to lift her into his arms and carry her across the great cold waters of death.

She sat in that heavenly embrace for what seemed to be a long time but in reality was only a minute or so.

She slowly dropped her arms and lay back in the bed, her head turned and eyes fixed on mine. I could not shift my eyes away from her fixed gaze.

I knew this was it. The time to say goodbye was now. As my heart was breaking, I watched the glow disappear from her face and the light of life in her eyes flicker dimly and finally go completely dark.

The look of life and love was now a lifeless stare of death. I didn't know what to do or say. She was gone.

I had other members of my family nearby but I felt so alone. Then another strange thing happened.

The doctors closed her eyes and

"officially" let us know she was gone.

There had been an abiding peace present in the room throughout the day which now took on a much more prominent role. God reminds us in His Word that the death of each of His saints is precious to Him.

The presence of Heaven was obvious and real in that room at that hour.

A spontaneous rendition of "Amazing Grace" swept across the room and down the hall.

As we said goodbye, Heaven said hello. We watched as Diana laid down her suffering, cancer-ravaged body.

Heaven watched her rise from the bed of affliction into the joy the Lord has prepared for those who love Him.

Suddenly, it was not a time of sadness but one of rejoicing. We knew it was not the end but only the beginning.

She could not return to us but we all could go to her. We would see her again.

One of the most traumatic times in life is the loss of a husband, wife, child, parent, sister, brother, grandparent or grandchild. Sometimes death comes suddenly, without warning. Other times it approaches like a slow-moving evening shadow. No matter how it arrives, death is always accompanied by a far-reaching, often devastating impact (Harris, 2009, p. 9).

With the case of a terminal illness, grief many times begins long before the actual death takes place.

Once death occurs, the caregiver moves into another period of transition in the caregiving process. The responsibilities of caregiving abruptly come to a halt and a time of refocusing of necessity begins.

Where do I go from here?

What Do I Do Now?

Dr. Paul Gentuso, our family practitioner and my personal friend checked for a heartbeat, pronounced Diana dead, and then closed her eyes. I vaguely remember signing some documents permitting Woodbine Funeral Home to take charge of her body.

The hospital room slowly began to empty. I made my way through the corridors, hallways, elevator and skywalk to the Baptist Hospital Parking Garage. I found my car and began driving home.

My three years of care giving had come to an abrupt end. What do I do now? I was not sure about how I should be feeling.

There was a sense of relief that swept

over me. I almost felt guilty. For the first time in three years I was no longer under tremendous pressure that had been there 24 hours a day, seven days a week, 365 days a year.

Later I came to understand that this was normal for people who were primary caregivers. For the past three years I was focused on providing my mate's every need.

My world was consumed with doctor visits, surgeries, chemotherapy treatments, radiation treatments, refilling prescriptions, making sure medications were taken at appropriate times, oxygen tanks were replenished and etc.

I prepared for bed not knowing what the future might hold. I didn't realize it at the time but I had entered into my second period of grief.

This was a transition moment. When a loved one passes on, the primary caregiver and those closest to him/her enter a different stage of grief. Anticipatory grief, the period that began with the realization that things would never be the same again and has now ended with the death of the loved one, comes to an end and a new stage of grief begins.

The second period of grieving may begin at any point during the transition stages of the anticipatory grief of caregiving and will come to a close when the grieving process has ended after the final stage of caregiving.

Period 1: Crisis and Shock

Crisis and shock are the initial emotional reactions to the death of a loved one or family member. This emotional reaction frequently includes panic, denial, shock and even disbelief at the loss of a loved one.

When one realizes that the family member is truly gone, the emotion of the moment is almost indescribable. Your whole world has suddenly turned upside down. You are almost numb and in a state of confusion.

You become emotionally drained and sometimes physically exhausted. This initial shock may last from a few minutes to several days.

How one reacts and behaves relating to circumstances and events may require revisiting later on in the grieving process. Sinful reactions should be mentally noted and dealt with later on.

False guilt is sometimes experienced during this shocking crisis time. Wishing one had done more for the loved one and feeling guilty. Remembering one specific incident or situation where one wishes he had said or done something differently. Regretting not being present at an important moment.

Feeling some guilt is normal. Sometimes there may be legitimate reasons. Remember, this feeling is normal and is birthed by the enormous emotional pain at the loss of a loved one.

I'll deal with this in more detail in the next chapter.

False blame sometimes surfaces during this time of crisis and shock. We strike out at others because of the pain we are experiencing. I'll talk more about this in the next chapter.

Unkind words to others may also be spoken. We become angry because of the pain of loss and strike out at others. I'll deal with this also in the next chapter.

Who Can I Blame?

I awoke with my bedside phone ringing. I glanced at the alarm clock while reaching for the phone and realized it was 2 o'clock in the morning.

My pastoral experience immediately caused a red flag; I knew this was probably not going to be good. The voice on the other end informed me that a two-year-old girl from our church had been taken to the emergency room.

I immediately dressed and drove to the hospital. Pastors in our small town were well known to hospital personnel. I was recognized and ushered through the double doors to the treatment rooms in the ER.

I was confronted with a scene that I will never forget. Susie (not her real name) was a

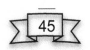

two-year-old beautiful little blond headed girl. Her mother checked on her in the middle of the night and found her not breathing.

They rushed her to the hospital and I arrived moments later. The family gathered in the family counseling room where I joined them.

John (the grandfather and not his real name) began describing the events taking place. Susie and her mother were living with Susie's grandparents. Susie's mother had become pregnant by a man who was married to another woman. The man was in the midst of divorce proceedings when he died suddenly in an automobile accident.

Susie's mother was devastated but our church wrapped their arms around her and adopted Susie as one of our own.

I sat quietly, intently listening as John gave me the details of what had happened. The doctor came into the room and closed the door. *I'm sorry, but there was nothing we could do. Susie passed away.*

Susie's mother collapsed and her grandfather began cursing and screaming at me. *What kind of God would kill my two-year-old granddaughter? That is not a God of love and I want nothing to do with him.*

I knew there was no point in responding to John's accusations at that moment. Days later he apologized to me for the way he treated me and for some of the things he'd said to me.

False Guilt - false blame and unkind words are very common when one experiences the loss of a loved one. One important thing to remember is that one may have to revisit some of those statements and unkind words and ask forgiveness after the reality of all that is happening sets in.

False guilt can lead to depression and spiritual paralysis. During the shocking loss of a close family member, we sometimes feel needless guilt.

Our minds may remind us of cross words we exchanged with our love ones. We feel guilty and wish we hadn't said those things.

We may remember something they had requested we were not able to provide at the time and feel guilty.

We wish we had called or visited them more often.

There are many reasons why false guilt seems to pervade our hearts and minds at the loss of the loved one.

A great principle to remember that helped me greatly is that we cannot undo the past. We are living in the present and how we live today may affect our future possibility for happiness.

If we realize there are issues that are reasons for feeling guilty, then we should ask God to forgive us knowing that we cannot change what has taken place. We must genuinely repent and ask for forgiveness. He will forgive us and then we must move on.

In most cases, the guilt is false. We did our very best to provide the care that our loved one needed. Sometimes even at the point of exhaustion we loved them and gave of ourselves.

We must try to remember that the overwhelming feelings of loss are contributing greatly to our guilty feelings.

We must remember that our loved ones would not want us to feel guilty. They would want us to remember how much we helped them during this most difficult time in their lives.

False Blame - blaming others for the loss of our loved ones sometimes happens during this time of shock at the initial loss of our loved ones. The pain hurts so badly that we want to blame someone.

We may blame the doctors, nurses, other family members, and hospital or special care facilities. Granted on occasion there is negligence on behalf of others and that must be addressed, but in most cases, others are not to blame. One good principle to remember is that God has his plan for each of us. When he chooses to take one of our loved ones he always knows what he is doing.

God is ultimately in control. He knew when and where we would be born and also knows when, where and how we will die. He knows those things about our loved ones as well.

So we must trust in the Lord even as Job did in Job 13:15: *Though he slay me, yet will I trust in Him*. We should remember that when it comes to God's children, anything that happens to us is always for our good and His glory in the end.

Unkind words - another important thing to remember is that we tend to strike out at those who are closest to us. When the sudden shock of losing a loved one strikes close to home, the emotion of the moment may manifest itself in harsh words toward those who care most for us.

We probably recognize what we've done as soon as the words leave our lips. We are hurt and angry and we may not feel like making things right at that moment.

But we should make a mental note and things should be made right at some point in the future after the initial shock has subsided.

This period of shock and crisis is a difficult time. But the important thing to remember is that this will pass. When one is in the middle of it that statement may seem distant and hard to believe.

Remember this wonderful principle found in the book of Lamentations 3:22-23a; *the steadfast love of the Lord never ceases, His mercies never come to an end; they are new every morning.*

God is with you and loves you more than you can imagine. His love is steadfast and never ceases. His grace is with you and just as the sun rises each morning, his promises are true every day.

One thing that helped me during this most difficult period was the sun rising in the morning after one of the most difficult nights in my life.

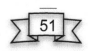

The sun has become a symbol for me. Each morning when the sun rises, I am reminded that God's promises are true. When you see the sun come up in the morning, remember that His promises that were true yesterday are also true today.

Another important principle to remember is to live life one day at a time. Yesterday is gone and tomorrow will always become today.

Ask God to help you make it through today. Don't worry about tomorrow, next week, next month or next year.

Here is a great passage of Scripture that might be helpful during this difficult period of time. Psalm 121:1-3; *I will lift up my eyes to the hills, from where my help comes. My help comes from the LORD, who made heaven and the earth. He will not suffer my foot to be moved: he that takes care of me will not sleep.*

World Upside Down

The funeral at Woodbine Free Will Baptist Church in Nashville was a time of rejoicing and celebration.

The graveside service at Harris Chapel Free Will Baptist Church was truly one to remember. The wonderful meal provided by the Cookeville church was a blessing.

We slowly began going our separate ways and my life turned in another direction.

The day had been a full one. I spent the night at my parent's home in Cookeville, TN. I dreaded returning to my home in Smyrna, Tennessee, knowing the house would be empty and I would be all alone.

I remember entering the house with a terrible sense of emptiness and loss. I knew my life had changed, but little did I know that my whole world had been turned upside down.

I moved beyond the crisis and shock of the death of my wife, and was now entering the period I later found out was called *disorganization*.

Disorganization is a very vulnerable time for grievers. It will last at least for weeks and could last several months.

Old life patterns and routines are forever altered and a time of chaos and confusion sets in. There is much to be said for routine. But when one loses a loved one, especially a spouse, their lifestyle has to change.

Living alone is much different than having a partner, best friend, and confidant with you. Do not be surprised with the sense of loneliness that you encounter. Unfortunately, this is part of the grieving process.

While sitting alone at home you may see something on TV and turn to speak to the loved one who is no longer there. You may be out and think *I'm going to be late I should call*

home only to remember no one is at home.

You may walk into your closet and catch the aroma of your loved one's cologne, perfume or aftershave and find yourself breaking into tears.

Activities with others will be different. You may find your relationship with close friends changes because you don't have as much in common with the passing of your loved one. You may feel like a fifth wheel because now you are alone with others who are couples.

The routine, time, etc. of eating meals will change. I found myself picking up food from restaurants and bringing it home to eat. Eating alone in a crowded room with many people was not a pleasant experience for me.

Responsibilities and tasks that your loved one once took care of now will fall to you. Handling finances, doing laundry, going to the grocery, repairs to the house, getting the car serviced, and etc. may now be your responsibility.

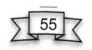

This time the grieving process can become overwhelming. Don't hesitate to talk to others, especially those who have already gone through the grieving process.

There are a number of grief support groups available that can be a tremendous help. You may want to consider becoming part one of those groups

It might be wise to consider talking with your pastor or a Christian counselor if you're having a difficult time coping.

The past may surface and a review of old patterns and things said and done during the crisis and shock period may need to be addressed. Forgiveness from God and others should be sought.

Making hasty decisions should be avoided. Be very careful about making decisions that could cause you to forfeit future happiness.

I would suggest not making major life-changing decisions for a period of one year. Some would suggest shorter periods of time and others longer periods of time. One year allows you time to move through a good portion of the grieving process.

Your head will be much clearer and you will have a greater sense of direction after 12 months or so. Other decisions will need to be made sooner, but be careful about stating what you will never do or what you are going to do.

Statements like *I'll never sell this house* might handcuff you in a way that your loved one would never have wanted. Be careful not to try and establish a monument to your loved one.

Widows have a hard time taking care off large houses and yards. Sometimes it makes much more sense to downsize into something that is more manageable.

We say we will never do this or that because we fear a sense of being disloyal to our loved.

Those who are grieving must be careful during this time. Great care should be given

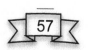

not to make quick decisions or binding statements.

Statements and decisions made during this time of disorganization can result in forfeiting any opportunity for future happiness.

Be careful about declaring that you will never marry again. The one flesh relationship is a powerful one designed by God himself. Remember your commitment was *till death parted you*.

Making the statement, I will never marry again, may cause you to live alone for the rest of your life. You were faithful to your mate when he/she was alive and you may feel that you are being unfaithful if you entertain the thought of falling in love again.

You will always have a place in your heart for the loved one that passed and no one will ever take that person's place. It's like when a new child is born into the family. He or she does not take the place of the other children, but parents make room in their hearts and love each one God gives.

That's exactly what could happen in your life. God might bless you with someone else who will love you and become your best friend. Do not limit God's intended happiness for you by closing the door on possible future happiness.

Do not say *I will never take this ring off.* I'm not saying that you should take your wedding ring off immediately after the passing of your loved one, but it is important not to make decisions during this time of disorganization that may hinder your future happiness. I'll talk more about the ring in another chapter.

One must also be careful in saying what he or she is going to do. Statements like *I'm selling this house and moving to Florida* may push you into a decision that you could regret later.

One other important factor may come into play during this period of time.

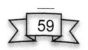

Sometimes one might feel guilty in accepting a life insurance payment when a loved one passes on.

There are a couple of things that it might be wise to remember. First, some expenses surrounding the illness and death of a loved one will not surface for weeks or months after their passing. You may need that money to address those bills and take care of unforeseen expenses.

Second, there is absolutely nothing wrong with accepting life insurance payments. Keep in mind that premium payments for the life insurance may have been made for many years. Those payments were made for such a time as this.

One should never feel guilty for receiving from what they have paid. Sometimes a mistake is made in saying *I cannot keep this money*.

The family income may decrease by 50% or more when a loved one dies. Life insurance was purchased to help with what follows after a loved one passes on. You may need the life insurance money to supplement your loss of income.

A great Bible principle to remember during this time of this disorganization is that God promises to give you direction. The Bible says in Psalm 37:23 *that a person's steps are made secure by the Lord when they delight in his way.*

Trust in the Lord with all your heart and he will give you a sense of direction and help you make important decisions (Proverbs 3:5-6 my paraphrase).

Dr. Roy W. Harris

Time to Reorganize

I remember reading a poem titled: *A Road Less Traveled*. It came at a dark and difficult time. I do not remember much about the words, but I identified with the concept.

The journey was so dark at times. I remember when I had prayed hard and fervently that God would heal and restore Diana. I almost became numb.

I felt so beaten down and battered by life that prayer became more difficult. Many times in the last months of Diana's life, I could only find words to beg God to help us.

Diana slept most of the time and I felt so alone. The chemo and cancer had affected her personality. I attended to her every need as best I could but she was not herself. She couldn't help it and I knew it.

She wanted to get a puppy. We'd had other dogs through the years, but I knew with her low resistance that it would not be a good idea. I knew also I just could not take on anything more and a puppy would require much time and attention. I remember her saying, "I want to get a puppy because I want something to need me."

My heart ached. Oh, how I needed her. Oh how I longed for a gentle word or a loving touch. She did not realize how it sounded. At that point she was so sick she no longer could see much of what was going on in my personal world.

It is hard to believe she is gone. Her struggle is over and her victory is assured. But how can one go on? Those were dark days and I could not understand how the sun could continue to rise in the morning.

I was not suicidal, but I wanted the Lord to just take me too. I was alone. Sure, I had family, friends and my church family, but no one was there when I came home at night. There was no longer a need to call home when I was going to be late. The emptiness was beyond description.

Carrying my own grief and shouldering the problems my church members faced were almost overwhelming at times. I had no one at home to support me or look after me.

I remember one day in particular. It was our anniversary. It had been nine months since Diana's death and Christmas was a week away. I remember visiting her grave and weeping. It had been nine months and the pain should have been less. How could I face Christmas alone?

God did a work in my heart that day as I laid two-dozen roses on the grave. He reminded me that He still had work for me to do. He had a plan for my life just as he had a plan for Diana's life.

I didn't hear an audible voice. The men in white coats may come and get you if you acknowledge that. But it was as though He was telling me: *Roy, you've had almost a year now. You've made it through all the firsts except for a couple more. You've made it through Mother's Day, Father's Day, your birthday, her birthday, and Thanksgiving. Souls are at risk and I have things for you to do. You must go on. You do have a life and this sad time will pass. You have followed me faithfully your entire adult life. I have not left you. I have not forsaken you. I have been faithful to you.*

Look at what you have around you. Look at your blessings. I have blessed you physically. You are healthy and have many years to live. I've blessed you personally.

You have two wonderful children who have fine Christian mates. You had three precious grandchildren before Diana's death and I have given you another one during your time of grief.

I've blessed you materially. Look at where you live, what you wear, how well you

*eat and what you drive. I've even gone the
extra mile and given you a Harley Davidson
motorcycle to ride (just kidding).*

*Look at how I've blessed you
spiritually. You have a great church and
you've had great opportunities of service
during your entire ministry.*

God was letting me know that it was
wrong for me to continue to focus on the hurt
and the grief. I could no longer continue to
stay in this state of sadness. Diana would not
have wanted it. My children did not want it.
But most importantly, God did not want it. I
talked to the Lord a great deal that day.

I made a decision that with His help, I
would do my best to move forward with my
life. I would find the future by looking for Him
in the present. I determined that I would work
on moving forward with my life one day at a
time. I had spent the last almost four years
taking life as it had come one day at a time. I
could see a light.

Time to Reorganize

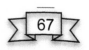

Some people never make it to this stage in the grieving process. They never make a conscious decision to move forward with their lives.

I've talked with people who allowed themselves to sink deeper and deeper into disorganized grief. They couldn't seem to get past the disruption the death of a loved one brings.

A period of reorganization is absolutely necessary if one is to survive and thrive through the grieving process. This period will last for several weeks but will possibly open the door for future direction and happiness.

The first step in the reorganization process is to make up your mind that you must move forward. This decision is not an easy one because it will require many changes.

Change has already begun because of the disorganized state one is thrust in after the passing of a loved one. We have no choice but to make changes.

This period of reorganization may last for several months. It will be characterized by reorganizing a number of things in one's life.

Let me mention a few things that I hope will be helpful. I remember talking with someone whose mother had passed away. They related to me how the mother had died at the kitchen table while drinking a cup of coffee.

The father refused to allow the cup and saucer to be removed from the table. It sat there for months. It was the last thing she had touched before she died and he would not let anyone remove it.

My daughter and daughter-in-law cleaned up my kitchen, cleaned out my refrigerator and rearranged a number of things in the kitchen. That needed to happen!

They discovered food that had been in my refrigerator for several months and was well past the time of safe eating. They also made my kitchen more accessible to me.

One mistake sometimes made by those

who've lost loved ones is trying to preserve things exactly the way they were before the loved one died. They want everything left in the exact place and nothing to be rearranged or changed. This is an impossible task.

Granted, some things are sentimental and have special meaning and should be kept and preserved. But other things of necessity need to be adjusted, rearranged or removed.

Months passed and I would find myself standing in my closet weeping. I finally realized what was triggering those emotions. My wife's clothes still hung neatly in the closet the way they were the night she passed away.

Each time I entered the closet I would smell her perfume and immediately my overwhelming grief would return. I recognized that I needed to do something with my closet situation.

I talked with my daughter and daughter-in-law and asked them if they would help me. I didn't feel that I could handle the finality of removing her clothes and seeing the closet mostly empty.

They both agreed to help me. I made plans to be away for the weekend and the two of them came over and went through my wife's clothes. They selected clothes that had special meaning for them and took them home. They donated the rest to an organization where other ladies would get good use from them.

I returned home after the weekend to find my closet completely rearranged. It seemed a little strange and took some getting used to, but I was so thankful that I'd overcome this huge hurdle.

There were three great benefits from our efforts of working together. First, I could move in and out of my closet without being emotionally paralyzed.

Second, the girls were able to select clothes that were special to them and they enjoyed wearing. This was a benefit to me also because I would recognize the clothes as Diana's when they wore them and it would bring a smile to my face.

Third, others would benefit from wearing her clothes rather than just leaving them closed up in the closet. I'm sure that's the way she would've wanted it.

What about wedding rings? Months had passed and I continued wearing my wedding band. After all, we had been married for 33 years and wearing my wedding band was a regular part of my wardrobe.

Eventually I decided it was time to remove the ring. I didn't put it in a drawer or place it out of my sight. I placed the wedding band on my key ring. I continue to see it each time I started my car or unlocked my front door.

This was important because I still had the rest of my life ahead of me. My wife was gone and was never returning. This didn't mean that I loved her less! But I remembered what she told me a few weeks before she died. She told me that she did not want me to be alone. She encouraged me to try and find happiness after she was gone.

I didn't want to hear those words as she was speaking them, but I'm so glad she spoke them in such a way that they continued with me long after her death.

Removing the wedding band from my finger was the first step toward opening a door to possible future happiness. I had no idea of the wonderful future God had planned for me.

You are not being disloyal or violating your wedding vows by removing your wedding band after your loved one has passed on. You are merely taking an important step to make possible your future happiness.

This may be the time to consider selling one of your vehicles or downsizing your home. It may be time to give some things to your children. This might be a good time to have a large yard sale and dispose of some things.

Reorganization is a necessary part of the grieving process. One has no choice but to rearrange and reorganize. Circumstances and

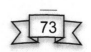

73

life situations demand it.

How we approach reorganization is of paramount importance. We must make up our minds that it is time to move forward.

One important biblical principle to remember is demonstrated by David in the Old Testament. Notice what David did when his son passed away and he received the news.

2 Samuel 12:19-20 says when David understood that the child was dead, he said to his servants, *"Is the child dead*?" They said, *"He is dead."* Then David arose from the earth and washed and anointed himself and changed his clothes. And he went into the house of the LORD and worshiped. He then went to his own house. And when he asked, they set food before him, and he ate.

David acted in one way before the child died and then reorganized his behavior after the child died.

We provide the best care we can for our loved ones. We are in serious emotional pain when we lose them. But there comes a point where we must make up our minds to allow God's plan to continue to unfold in our lives.

His plan was for our loved ones to go to Him and His plan for us is to continue to live lives that bring honor and glory to Him.

We must make up our minds to say yes to whatever God has in store for us. We must open the door to our future by closing the door on our past.

It's time to reorganize, rearrange and reset our priorities for the future.

What Should I Expect?

Coping with grief begins with becoming aware of what may come your way during this transition in the grief journey. Dr. Therese Rando in her book *How To Go on Living When Someone You Love Dies* provides great practical insight into what might be expected during the grieving process in her section called *Grief: Appropriate Expectations* (Rando, 1991, pp. 79-80). Knowing what one might expect can be a tremendous help in transitioning through the grieving process.

Below is a list of practical observations of what one might expect during his/her time of grief.

1. Your grief may take *longer* than you think.

2. Your grief may take *more energy* than you might have imagined.

3. Your grief may involve *many changes* and be *continually developing*.

4. Your grief may *show itself* in *all spheres* of your life including psychological, social and physical.

5. Your grief may *depend* on how you *perceive* the loss.

6. You may grieve for *many things* both *symbolic* and *tangible*, not just the death alone.

7. You may grieve for what you have *already lost* and for what you have also *lost in the future*.

8. Your grief may entail *mourning* not only for the actual person lost but *also* for all of the *hopes*, *dreams* and *unfulfilled expectations* you held for and with that person, and for the *needs* that may go *unmet* because of the death.

9. Your grief may *involve* a wide variety of *feelings* and *reactions*, not solely those that are generally thought of as grief, such as *depression* and *sadness*.

10. Your loss may *resurrect* old *issues*, *feelings* and *unresolved conflicts* from the past.

11. You may have some identity confusion as a result of this major loss and the fact that you are experiencing reactions that may be quite different.

12. You may have a combination of anger, depression, irritability, frustration, annoyance or intolerance.

13. You may feel anger and guilt or at least some manifestation of these emotions.

14. You may have a lack of self-concern.

15. You may experience grief spasms, acute upsurges of grief that occur suddenly with no warning.

16. You may have trouble with thinking, memory, organization, intellectual processing and making decisions. You

may feel like you are going crazy.

17. You may be obsessed with the death and preoccupied with the deceased.

18. You may begin a search for meaning and may question your religion and/or philosophy of life.

19. You may find yourself acting socially in ways that are different from before.

20. You may find yourself having a number of physical reactions.

21. You may find that there are certain dates, events, and stimuli that bring surges in grief.

22. Society may have unrealistic expectations about your mourning and may respond inappropriately.

23. Certain experiences later in life may resurrect intense grief temporarily.

This list gives a great overview of possible things one might experience during the grieving process. It also gives insight into possible misconceptions and alerts you to identify what may come your way.

I would encourage you to review the individual items on the list occasionally while within the walls of grief. This may help reassure you that the feelings you are experiencing are not uncommon and are normal.

There is a combination of factors that impact grief. Those who are grieving should become aware that their grief brings an intense amount of emotion that will surprise them and those around them.

Grief will not only be more intense than they expected, but it will also manifest itself in more areas and ways than they anticipated.

They can expect brief upsurges of emotion for no apparent reason. These times remind them of what they have lost.

How those who are grieving cope

with grief will be depend greatly on how much they have lost, their personalities, the type death their loved one experienced, how much support they receive from family and friends and caregivers' physical health (Lachman, 2013).

Coping With Grief

Dr. Larry Lachman's article *Grief & Loss: Caring for the Caregiver after Death* offers a number of steps that can help not only former caregivers but also most people transition through the grieving process (Lachman, 2013).

Caregivers should be aware that it didn't take an hour to become close and connected with their recently departed loved one, so it will take more than an hour to get over the pain of their loss. The relationship they established with their spouses, parents or child took place over time. Likewise, the grief process and the painful feelings associated with it will also take time to resolve.

People grieve at different rates in different ways. There is no fixed way of grieving, including the six phases mentioned earlier. Caregivers should take their time. There is no ONE right way to grieve.

The most intense feelings of loss can take from one to three years to dissipate before emerging from the emotional abyss of grief.

Caregivers should keep in mind they will grieve as deeply as they loved. The more they loved someone, the deeper they will grieve.

Beware of reminders. When caregivers are grieving, almost anything and everything can remind them of their loved ones. Simple things like songs on the radio, smells at restaurants and favorite cereals at the supermarket to name a few.

Anniversaries, birthdays, Christmas, Thanksgiving, Mother's Day and Father's Day are typically the most difficult times a year for those who are grieving.

Caregivers should be prepared. It is absolutely normal to sink into the emotional abyss and feel deeply saddened, to feel pain and miss the person loved during these times. The first two years are the most difficult for getting through the holidays. Beginning with the third year, typically the pain becomes less painful; the sadness is a little less sad and the sobbing less intense.

When one of these significant holidays comes about, expect to take a step or two backwards for every step forward made in grief.

Grievers should surround themselves with supportive people. They should do what they need to do for their mind, body and spirit to ritualize and acknowledge their pain.

Those who are grieving sometimes idolize or demonize the person for whom they are grieving. The spouse or parent continues putting the deceased partner or child up on a pedestal as if they could do no wrong or they concentrate on all the bad and inconsiderate things that the person did while they were still alive.

Both of these tendencies are to protect the soul. These protective maneuvers reduce pain.

It's hard for a recently bereaved person to think about bad things their departed love one did when they were alive, without feeling pangs of guilt for thinking such thoughts.

However, by not doing this, it causes grievers to become out of balance and keeps them stuck in their grief.

Those who are grieving must work through fear of thinking anything negative about their departed loved one would be disrespectful in some way.

Sooner or later, they must be able to do this in order to fully let go and say good-bye to the person they've lost.

Similar dynamics are also true for those who demonize their lost loved one. It's always easier to say good-bye or let go of someone when angry and indignant instead of being hurt or feeling sad.

Our anger masks the pain and empowers us to say what we need to say and move on.

However, anger is a secondary emotion, which is fueled by two other primary emotions: hurt and fear.

These feelings frequently arise from the shadow side of our emotions. Until those feelings of hurt and fear are brought out and dealt with, grievers will not be able to move forward in their mourning process.

They must say good-bye and do this by looking at the whole person for whom they are grieving, both the good and the bad.

Caregivers in grief need to be aware that they will often come out of their experience of caretaking feeling like a battle-fatigued soldier returning from war.

In addition to normal feelings of grief, caregivers may experience symptoms of Post-Traumatic Stress Disorder, which includes: nightmares, flashbacks, depression, anxiety and avoiding all places, people and activities that were associated with the trauma of caregiving.

This is normal, but sometimes may have to

be dealt with in one-on-one therapy with a licensed psychologist familiar with treating PTSD.

Sometimes medication, twelve weeks or so, may be needed to help caregivers sleep and feel less depressed or anxious. These can be prescribed by family physicians or consulting psychiatrists.

Caregivers in grief who feel they may be suffering from PTSD should make an appointment with their physician or get a referral to a psychiatrist who can provide the proper medication needed.

Those who are grieving sometimes begin to feel lost as if they are like a ship without an anchor. They had defined themselves through familiar roles such being a wife, mother, or daughter. Once their husband, child or parent is gone, they now feel like they no longer have any roles. In essence, they feel role-less! They must find ways to find new roles.

They must redefine who they are by determining what they want out of life.

They must establish a new set of goals. This is a difficult process, but with time, sharing and bouncing ideas with others, they gradually develop their own new normal.

Grieving is fatiguing. Grievers should give themselves permission to be less than perfect.

They may not be able to do the things they normally did before their loss due to not enough energy to keep up with their current obligations.

Those who experience grief related fatigue often feel guilty for not being super mom, super husband or super human being. This is a difficult issue because it's connected with self-worth stemming from personal history and how much encouragement was given while they were growing up.

Many grievers were raised with the admonition to put other people's needs first rather than becoming self-absorbed or being selfish by tending to their own needs.

Lachman reminds grievers that they can only show others love, care and compassion if

they first have it for themselves. Grievers
must be okay with giving to themselves first,
before they can successfully give to others.
They must be willing to nourish their own lives
before they can help nourish someone else's.

They should remind themselves about all
that they sacrificed providing love and care for
their loved one and now it's time to allow
them to receive some of that very same care
from others while grieving.

A Moment of Revelation

Written below was written in an earlier chapter in the book, but I feel that it is worth repeating again as a moment for you to reflect on your future.

You must come to a moment like this and make that all-important decision to move forward with whatever God has in store for your future.

It is hard to believe she is gone. Her struggle is over and her victory is assured. But how can one go on?

Those were dark days and I could not understand how the sun could continue to rise in the morning.

I was not suicidal, but I wanted the Lord to just take me too. I was all alone. Sure, I had family, friends and my church family, but no one was there when I came home at night.

There was no longer a need to call home when I was going to be late. The emptiness was beyond description.

Carrying my own grief and shouldering the problems my church members were facing was almost overwhelming at times. I had no one at home to support me or look after me.

I remember one day in particular. It was our anniversary. It had been almost nine months since Diana's death and Christmas was a week away.

I remember visiting her grave and weeping. Even though it had been almost nine months, I felt that the pain should have been less. How could I face Christmas alone?

God did a work in my heart that day as I laid two-dozen roses on her grave. He reminded me that He still had work for me to do. He had a plan for my life just as he had a plan for Diana's life.

I didn't hear an audible voice. The men in

white coats may come and get you if you acknowledge that. But it was as though He was telling me:

Roy, you've had almost a year now. You've made it through all the firsts except for a couple more.

You've made it through Mother's Day, Father's Day, your birthday, her birthday, and Thanksgiving.

Souls are at risk and I have things for you to do. You must go on. You do have a life and this sad time will pass.

You have followed me faithfully your entire adult life. I have not left you. I have not forsaken you. I have been faithful to you.

Look at what you have around you. Look at your blessings. I have blessed you physically. You are healthy and have many years to live. I've blessed personally.

You have two wonderful children who have fine Christian mates. You had three precious grandchildren before

Diana's death and I have given you another one during your time of grief.

I've blessed you materially. Look at where you live, what you wear, how well you eat and what you drive.

Look at how I've blessed you spiritually. You have a great church and you've had great opportunities of service during your entire ministry.

God was letting me know that it was wrong for me to continue to focus on the hurt and the grief. I could no longer continue remaining in this state of sadness.

Diana would not have wanted it.

My children did not want it.

But most importantly, God did not want it.

I talked to the Lord a great deal that day. I made a decision that with His help, I would do my best to move forward with my life.

I would find the future by looking for Him in the present. I determined that I would work on moving forward with my life one day at a time.

I had spent the last almost four years taking life as it had come one day at a time.

The Final Chapter

God's rainbow was the beginning of many new and great things He would send my way.

He restored my joy.

He opened opportunities of service that have impacted thousands of lives.

Not so long ago I dreaded seeing the sunrise in the morning. Now I am excited about today and the future.

I haven't found the pot of gold at the end of the rainbow yet, but I have found a beautiful rainbow after a long, dark and violent storm.

I hear the birds singing again. I smell the pleasant fragrance of spring flowers and freshly cut grass. I notice the beautiful sunset.

Life is good. God is great. Will I ever

completely get over the experience of losing a close loved one? I doubt it.

The key is not trying to get completely over a tragic loss, but learning to live with and beyond it.

There is life after a great loss. One's own personal attitude greatly impacts what kind of life he will experience.

You can choose to remain in the grip of grief, pain and sorrow. It is not a great way to live. You will be miserable and make others who love and care about you sad and miserable also.

You do have a second choice. You can recognize there are people who love and need you. They need you happy and contented. They need you upbeat and positive. They need you present and engaged with their lives.

You can make up your mind that with God's help, you are going to move forward with your life.

God has a plan for you just as He did

for your dear loved one. It's His will for you
to have joy and to find your place in life.
Finding that plan begins with knowing Him
personally.

God has more in store for you.

You can *live through and beyond grief* and it is
God's will for you to do so.

Encouraging Scriptures

Psalm 46:1

"God is our refuge and strength, a very present help in trouble."

Hebrews 4:15-16

"For we do not have a High Priest who cannot sympathize with our weaknesses, but was in all points tempted as we are, yet without sin. Let us therefore come boldly to the throne of grace, that we may obtain mercy and find grace to help in time of need."

Hebrews 13:5-6

"For He has said, 'I will never leave you nor forsake you.' So we may boldly say: 'The LORD is my helper; I will not fear. What can man do to me?'"

Psalm 46:1-2

God is our refuge and strength, a very present help in trouble. Therefore we will not fear, Even though the earth is removed, And though the mountains be carried into the midst of the sea.

Peter 5:6-7

"Humble yourselves, therefore, under the mighty hand of God so that at the proper time he may exalt you, casting all your anxieties on him, because he cares for you."

Proverbs 3:5-6

"Trust in the LORD with all your heart, and lean not on your own understanding; in all your ways acknowledge Him, and He shall direct your paths."

Matthew 7:7

"Ask, and it will be given to you; seek, and you will find; knock, and it will be opened to you."

Romans 8:28

"And we know that for those who love God all things work together for good, for those who are called according to his purpose."

Isaiah 41:10

"Fear not, for I am with you; be not dismayed, for I am your God; I will strengthen you, I will help you, I will uphold you with my righteous right hand."

James 4:7

"Submit yourselves therefore to God. Resist the devil, and he will flee from you."

Philippians 4:6-7

"Do not be anxious about anything, but in everything by prayer and supplication with thanksgiving let your requests be made known to God. And the peace of God, which surpasses all understanding, will guard your hearts and your minds in Christ Jesus."

Psalm 23:1-6

A Psalm of David – "The Lord is my shepherd; I shall not want. He makes me lie down in green pastures. He leads me beside still waters. He restores my soul. He leads me in paths of righteousness for his name's sake. Even though I walk through the valley of the shadow of death, I will fear no evil, for you are with me; your rod and your staff, they comfort me. You prepare a table before me in the presence of my enemies; you anoint my head with oil; my cup overflows"

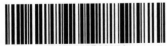

Made in the USA
Middletown, DE
18 September 2017